Intermittent Fasting and the Ketogenic Diet

The One/Two Punch

for

Lasting Weight Loss

Ron Kness

Published by:

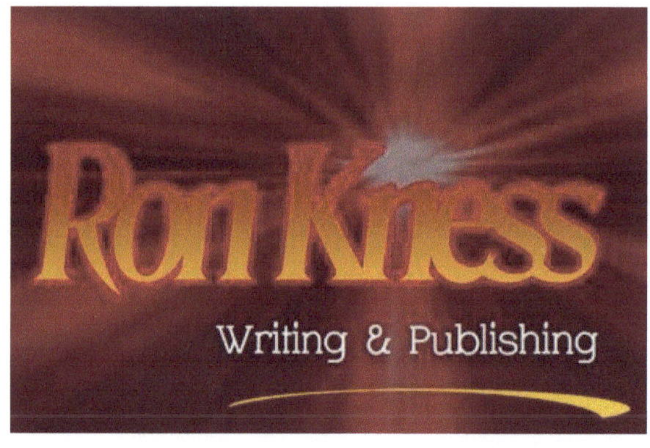

Ron Kness

San Tan Valley, AZ

United States of America

ISBN: 9781696044264

https://healthylifestylenewsletter.com

Sneak Peek

In my new book ***Intermittent Fasting and the Ketogenic Diet***, we combine two different eating styles together, and in doing so extract a synergy that individually they cannot create. While the keto diet is about *what* and *how much* you eat, intermittent fasting is about *when* you eat. By combining both together into a healthy-eating lifestyle, it is twice as effective. To get a better understanding of each eating style, let's look at each one individually.

Understanding the Keto Diet

You can't read a health or lifestyle blog or walk down an aisle in the grocery store without the words "keto diet" catching you eye these days. The low-carb/high-fat approach to eating has taken the country by storm and is creating quite a buzz for its ability to help you lose weight and burn fat. If you are considering a keto diet, then it is essential you learn not only the basics but the details about this approach to eating so that you can make the best choice for you.

The keto part of this guide explores everything you want to know about ketogenic eating, including what you can and can't eat for ketosis. We explore the health benefits as well as the precautions you should know, and we share some tips to help you make the most of your keto diet experience.

The ketogenic or keto diet is an eating plan that focuses on eating low-carb, high-fat foods. In addition to helping some people lose weight, it has other health benefits. The focus on the keto diet on low carb eating encourages your body to enter a state of ketosis, wherein it is using stored fat cells in your body for energy rather than the carbohydrates in your diet. Ketosis cannot be attained when there are already carbs for your body to use.

Looking at the basics of the keto diet, you want to strive for limited carbohydrates and more of your calories from fat – but not just any fat – the good fat. While we each process and metabolize food differently, the most common percentages touted among the keto community today is you should keep your intake of carbs under 50 grams per day, but stricter adherents recommend eating under 30 grams per day. Most people on a keto diet strive to eat 60 to 70 percent of their calories from fat, 15 to 30 percent from protein, and just 5 to 10 percent from carbs.

There are, however, several variations of the keto diet that you may want to consider, based on your needs. Some people do better with a cyclical keto diet, which includes five days of following a standard keto diet and two days of higher carb eating.

Other people choose to add in more carbs around workouts or physical activities. Some people believe that more protein is beneficial for them, so they choose a ratio that includes about 60 percent fat, 35 percent protein, and 5 percent carbs. There is little evidence to support the weight loss effects of some of these forms of ketogenic eating, as only the standard and higher protein versions have been much studied in the scientific literature.

Most of the people choosing to adopt a keto diet these days are doing so to lose weight. This type of eating plan is used under exceptional circumstances to manage specific medical conditions, such as epilepsy, but in general, it is not recommended that you follow a keto lifestyle for extended periods. In this guide, we explore some of the health benefits, but there is little evidence as to the long-term effects on eating for ketosis, except for continued weight management.

The ketogenic diet was initially developed to treat epilepsy and other types of seizure disorders. The ketones and decanoic acids produced by this way of eating both help to minimize seizures. Those who adhere to this eating plan, though, often experience weight loss, though. Eating carbohydrates provide your body with a ready source of energy, which means your cells never turn to your stored fat to help it perform its daily functions. Carbs also trigger cravings, which can lead to overeating, another source of weight gain.

As the buzz about the keto diet grew, more and more celebrities started following it, which caused it to catch fire among the general population. For many, eating the "keto way" is easy to follow and makes sense, which allows them to accomplish their weight loss goals.

One of the reasons that the keto diet often works, though, is that by merely focusing more intentionally on what you eat, you are more likely to eat less. People on any diet tend to reduce their caloric intake, at least for a while. Eating fats and proteins leads to feeling fuller faster, which can stop you from overeating, too. It also takes more energy for your body to process these macronutrients, versus carbs, so you are also burning more calories during digestion than you previously did. If looking for a two-week diet plan to get you started, you can get mine here at: https://forms.aweber.com/form/64/285395664.htm.

Most people on the keto diet lose between one and two pounds per week if they follow the plan carefully. Everyone is different, though, so you should not expect your results to be the same if your metabolic rate is slower or faster.

Your caloric needs may also differ if you are an athlete, perform physical work of any kind, or spend a lot of time outdoors. Keto eating will not help you lose weight if you are still eating too many calories. Reducing your intake is still necessary for the keto diet to result in weight loss.

Understanding Intermittent Fasting

Intermittent fasting or IF has taken the health and dieting world by storm over the past few years, with more and more followers sharing their remarkable journeys to improved weight loss. While many people try intermittent fasting to help shed excess pounds, others use it because of its health benefits or because of how it helps to simplify their lifestyle.

But what is intermittent fasting, and what exactly does it do to your body and mind? Those and many more questions are answered in this intermittent fasting portion of this guide. We explore the ins and outs of this way of eating, including what science tells us about how IF can help you lose weight, live longer, and think more clearly.

Intermittent fasting is basically a way of eating that requires you to go for more extended periods between eating and to consume food only within a prescribed, shorter window of time. There is no specific eating plan with IF, and you can use it with any type of meal plan, including keto, whole-foods, clean eating, or whatever floats your boat. Because it is not about WHAT foods you eat but instead WHEN you eat, it is not a traditional diet but could be looked at to improve your eating habits, no matter what you consume.

There are many variations to intermittent fasting, which we explore more in-depth below, but the most common window is referred to as 16:8, which means 16 hours of fasting while eating all your food for one day in an eight-hour window.

Fasting has been used across cultures for various purposes for thousands of years. While some types of fasting are forced, because of a lack of food, others are performed as a part of religious or ceremonial rituals. Our ancient predecessors were often without food during the hunter-gatherer phase of our evolution, so our bodies are conditioned to go without food for extended periods. It is only within the more abundant 20th century that people in our country began to expect and assume food to be available to them several times per day.

Our bodies would argue that fasting is more natural and optimal for its function than eating three or four times per day, and those who practice IF would agree. Many who choose this way of eating report improvements in their health beyond weight loss, and they continue to adhere to a fasting schedule long after they have reached their goal weight.

In this guide, we look at how combining both the keto diet and intermittent fasting is possibly the ideal healthy-eating plan.

Contents

Disclaimer

We hope you enjoy reading this publication; however, we do suggest you read our disclaimer.

All the material written in this document is provided for informational purposes only and is general in nature.

Every person is a unique individual and what has worked for some or even many may not work for you. Any information perceived as advice must be considered in light of your own particular set of circumstances.

The author or person sharing this information does not assume any responsibility for the accuracy or outcome of your use of the content.

Every attempt has been made to provide well researched and up to date content at the time of writing. Now all the legalities have been taken care of, please enjoy the content.

Introduction

The ketogenic diet has been in mainstream media for some time now, but the latest buzz is all about intermittent fasting, and when these two diet methods are done in tandem the results are greatly amplified.

If you're wanting a fat-burning surge to your keto lifestyle, intermittent fasting might be just what you need.

Intermittent fasting and the ketogenic diet are well known for their weight loss benefits, and others too, if followed correctly. Intermittent fasting leads to a number of changes in the body making it easier to burn fat and to help boost your metabolism.

When you consume food, your body uses the energy from these foods as fuel. During fasting periods your body is not consuming foods, so it will resort to using your stored fat as fuel.

This effect results in fat burning and weight loss.

In recent studies it has been shown that 84% of people who participate in any type of intermittent fasting not only lose weight, but they lose weight faster than the people who go on a low carbohydrate diet.

While participating in fasting regimes there is also some evidence that you will hold onto more muscle mass than you would while following most weight loss diets.

What is Intermittent Fasting?

Fasting has been around for centuries. Greek philosophers advocated fasting for medical purposes. Spiritual fasting is said to enhance purification and act as a form of soul cleansing. And metabolically speaking, your body has two phases: fed and fasted.

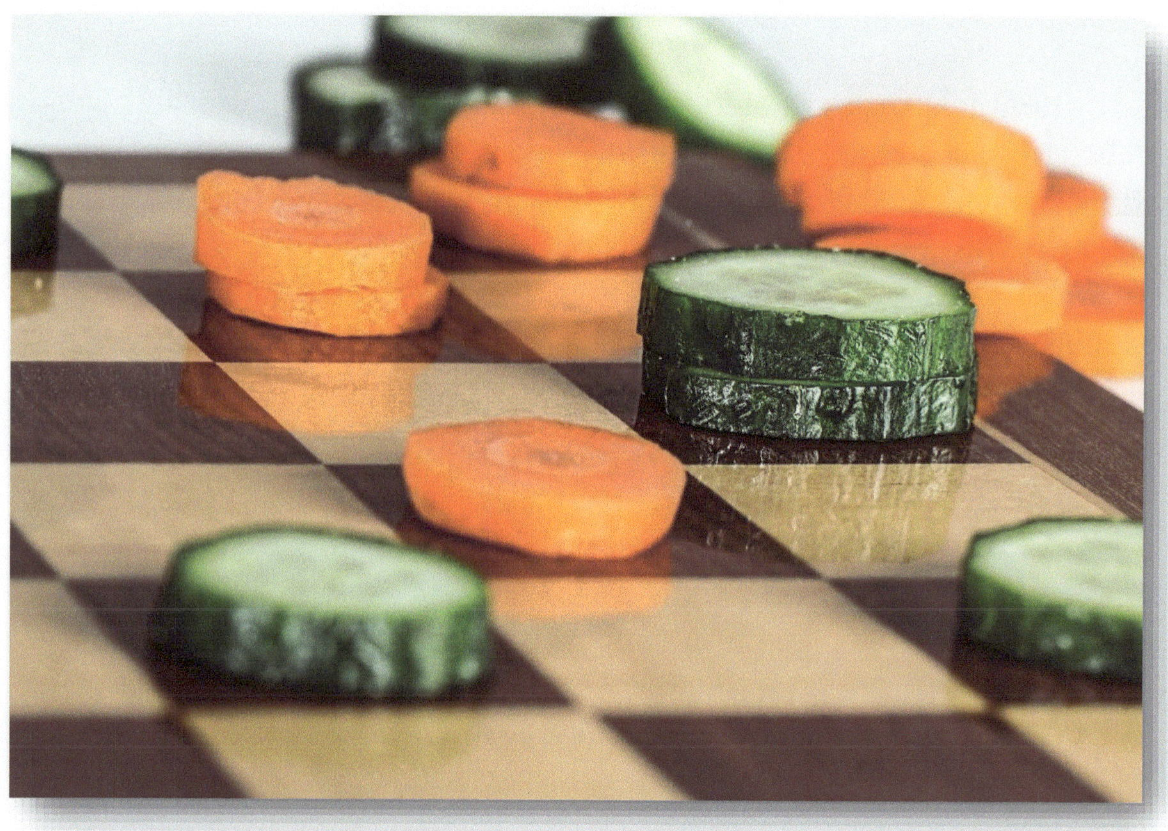

If you are one of the millions who tends to skip breakfast, you're already fasting and probably didn't even realize it.

The main concept behind intermittent fasting is *when* you eat and not necessarily *what* you eat – the later being the basis behind the Keto diet. There are several methods for this way of eating, the most common being a daily window, or timeframe, where eating is allowed.

If your "feeding" window is a 6-hour timeframe from noon to 6pm, your intermittent fasting ratio would be 18/6. The window is adjustable to suit your needs and typically somewhere between three to eight hours.

During the fasting phase, don't freak out! You won't starve. In fact, drinking things like bone broth, water, plain tea and plain coffee are permissible in the fasting phase, and are great to avoid dehydration. Avoid snacking though. The idea is to fast until feeding time.

When it's time to eat, there is a little planning necessary. The goal is to consume all of your daily calories in whatever window of time you've chosen for the feeding phase of your intermittent fast.

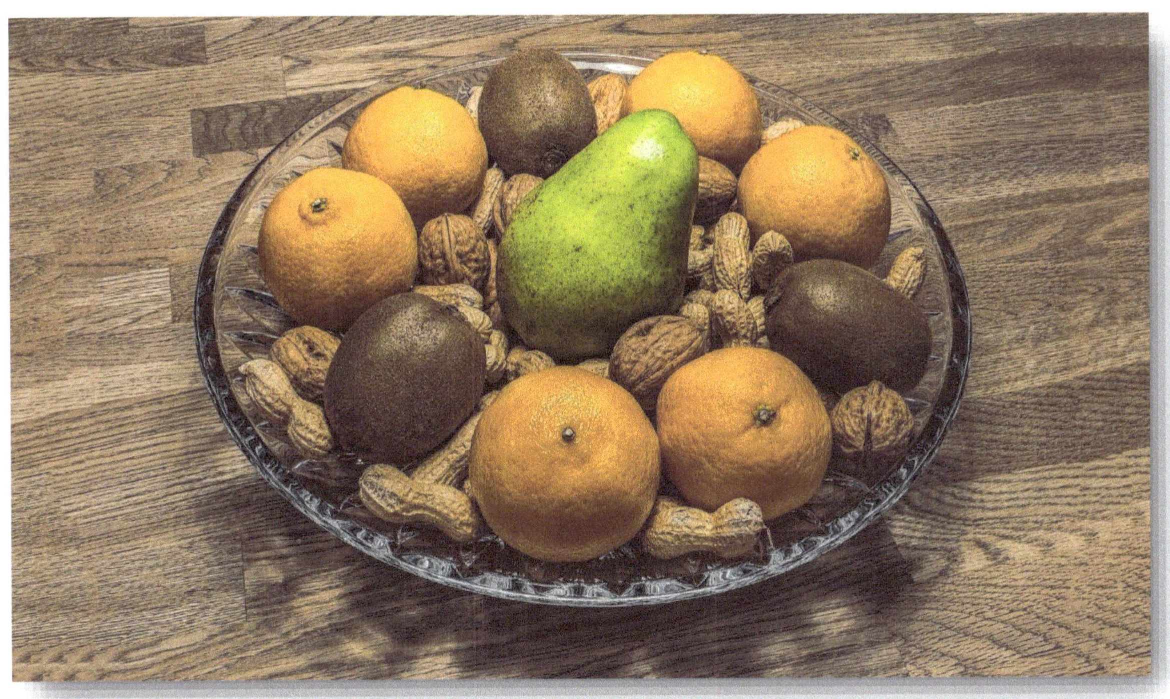

What is Ketosis?

When glucose is available, the body will draw on it first to provide the fuel for its energy requirements. Glucose which is excess to needs will eventually be converted to fat storage, so the body can draw on these reserves in time of prolonged food shortage.

In our modern, civilized environment, this is a fairly rare occurrence.

Ketosis is a completely normal metabolic state that happens when immediate reserves of glucose have been depleted, ideally (for the purpose of bodyfat reduction and blood glucose balancing) as a result of reduced carbohydrate intake.

When you are fasting or restricting carbs your body naturally moves to the next available source of energy, which are ketones, derived from stored fats. In the absence of glucose, the body switches over to burning fat for energy.

For someone wanting to reduce bodyfat, or to help reduce blood glucose levels, this is a desirable state for the body to be in.

Due to our physiology, the body is reluctant to burn bodyfat, as we have evolved to be prepared for some possible future dearth or famine. This means that simply missing out on a meal here and there will not cause your body to enter a state of ketosis and start burning fat.

If have entered a ketonic state, consuming too many carbohydrates, or virtually any simple carbohydrates, which are excess to the body's immediate energy requirements, will 'switch off' ketosis and put the body back into fat storage mode.

Anyone who is trying to attain and maintain a state of ketosis needs to become aware of their macronutrient (fats, proteins and carbs) requirements. This is to enable ketosis, and also to ensure essential nutrition needs are met.

This can vary from person to person depending on both lifestyle (such as work and exercise) and physiological factors (such as metabolic rates) Each person may need some experimentation to determine the ideal ratio for their goals and health status.

As a starting point, the generally recommended macronutrient percentages are:

- 5-10% of daily calories from carbohydrates
- 15-30% of daily calories from protein
- 60% or more of daily calories from fat

For the great many individuals who have for decades been led to believe that dietary fat is evil, the recommended fat levels can be confronting. Just remember, dietary fat is not the same as bodyfat, and the body converts simple carbohydrates to bodyfat far more easily.

So, no more wasted time looking for '97% fat-free' products, in fact these are almost always to be avoided when trying to achieve ketosis.

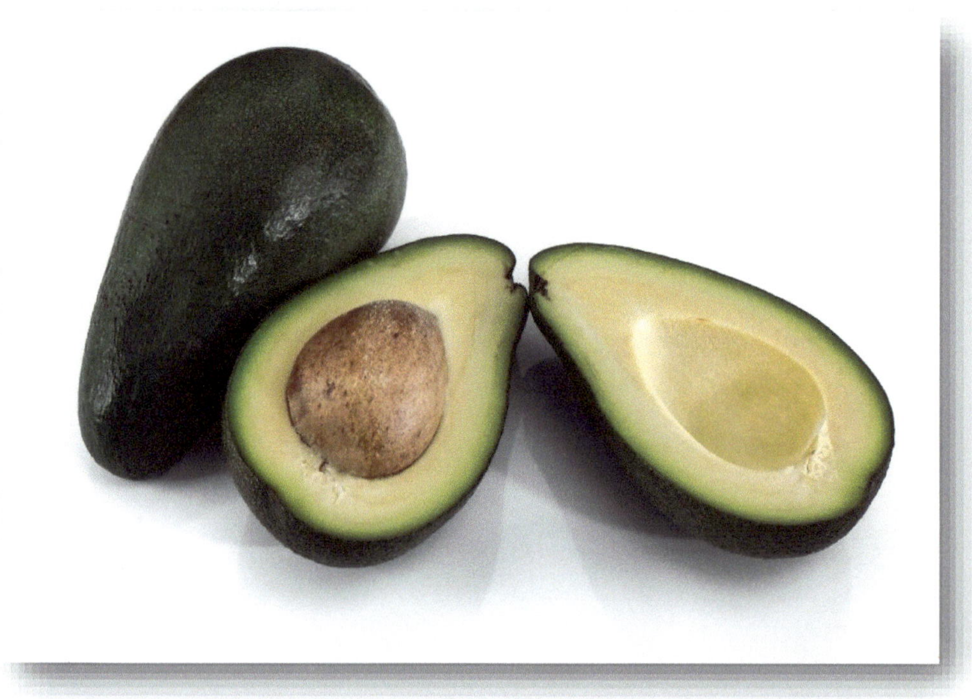

Three Popular Intermittent Fasting Methods for Weight Loss

One of the most popular versions of intermittent fasting is the '16/8' method.

There are two other popular intermittent fasting methods, the 'Eat-Stop-Eat' and the '5:2 Diet'.

16/8 Fasting Method

The '16/8' method is a non-fasting (eating permitted) period of 8 hours followed by 16 hours of fasting. Generally non-fasting is undertaken between the hours of 11am – 7pm.

This is partly to make it easier to align mealtimes with non-dieting others, but also due to this being the higher energy requirement time. Nocturnal eating is not conducive to helping achieve reduced bodyfat levels.

Eat-Stop-Eat Fasting Method

The 'Eat-Stop-Eat' method consists of doing one or two 24-hour periods of complete fasting each week, for example in the one x 24-hour period, you would eat breakfast one day and then eat nothing until breakfast again the next day.

In the two x 24 period scenario, you would eat breakfast, refrain from eating the rest of that day and all the next, and then eat breakfast the following (third) day.

5:2 Fasting Method

The 5:2 diet involves eating 500 - 600 calories two days of the week and eating normally the other 5 days. As long as healthy foods are consumed during the non-fasting periods weight loss should be achieved.

Can You Intermittently Fast and Follow the Keto Diet at The Same Time?

The short answer is yes. Both are diets. Both are extremely effective. And both share one major component - ketosis.

If intermittent fasting and the ketogenic diet are teamed up and used in tandem, they create quite a powerful duo – the one/two punch to lasting weight loss.

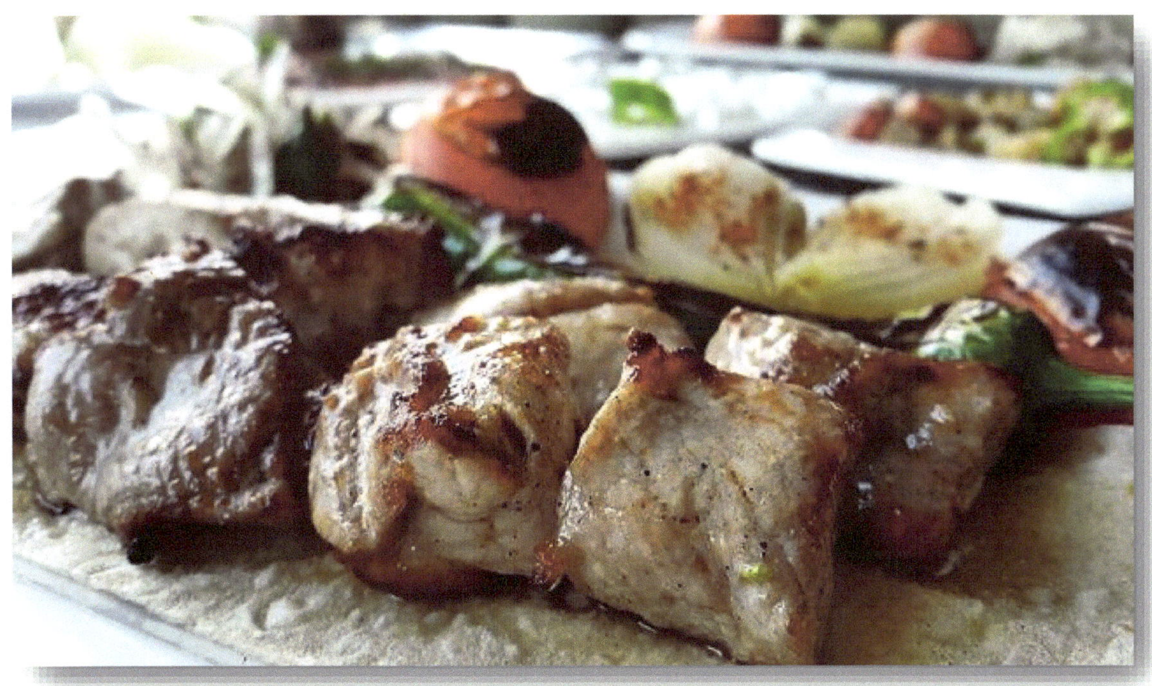

To get the big picture and fully understand how both diets work even better together, it's important to know the basics on how they work on a solo level.

Intermittent Fasting as a Way of Eating

From a metabolic standpoint, the human body has two states: fed and fasted. Intermittent fasting, in the most basic sense, is centered on *when* you eat instead of *what* you eat. At first glance, it sounds like a fluke.

There's no way that could work to lose weight or improve health! You would be starving yourself!

Untrue. Intermittent fasting actually pushes the body into a state of ketosis, which, if you're not yet on the keto diet bandwagon, enables the body to use stored fat for energy versus using carbohydrates. There are all sorts of ways to engage in intermittent fasting, but we will just look at the three most common:

1. *Fasting for a Meal* – Regularly skip a meal, any meal. It doesn't matter what meal, but for an overnight fast you'd probably choose skipping dinner or breakfast.

2. *Fasting for Hours* – Eat only during a specific window of time. You could fast for 20 hours and have a 4-hour window of opportunity to eat.

3. *Fasting for Days* – No eating for a specified number of days during the week and then resume eating normally for the remaining days.

When food is restricted glucose availability declines. Your body must find an alternate fuel. This is when ketosis begins. Ketones will now be the source of energy.

Another, often unexpected, benefit of intermittent fasting is smaller portions needed to achieve 'feeling full'. You might feel as hungry as a baseball team of teenage boys in a buffet line, but you're more likely to stop eating when you're sated.

https://healthylifestylenewsletter.com

The Keto Diet as a Way of Eating

For the ketogenic diet to be effective, carbohydrates are restricted while fats and proteins are increased. Again, the purpose here is to force the body into a state of ketosis so stored fats are used for energy instead of sugars/glucose, which is the reason for the strict carb limit.

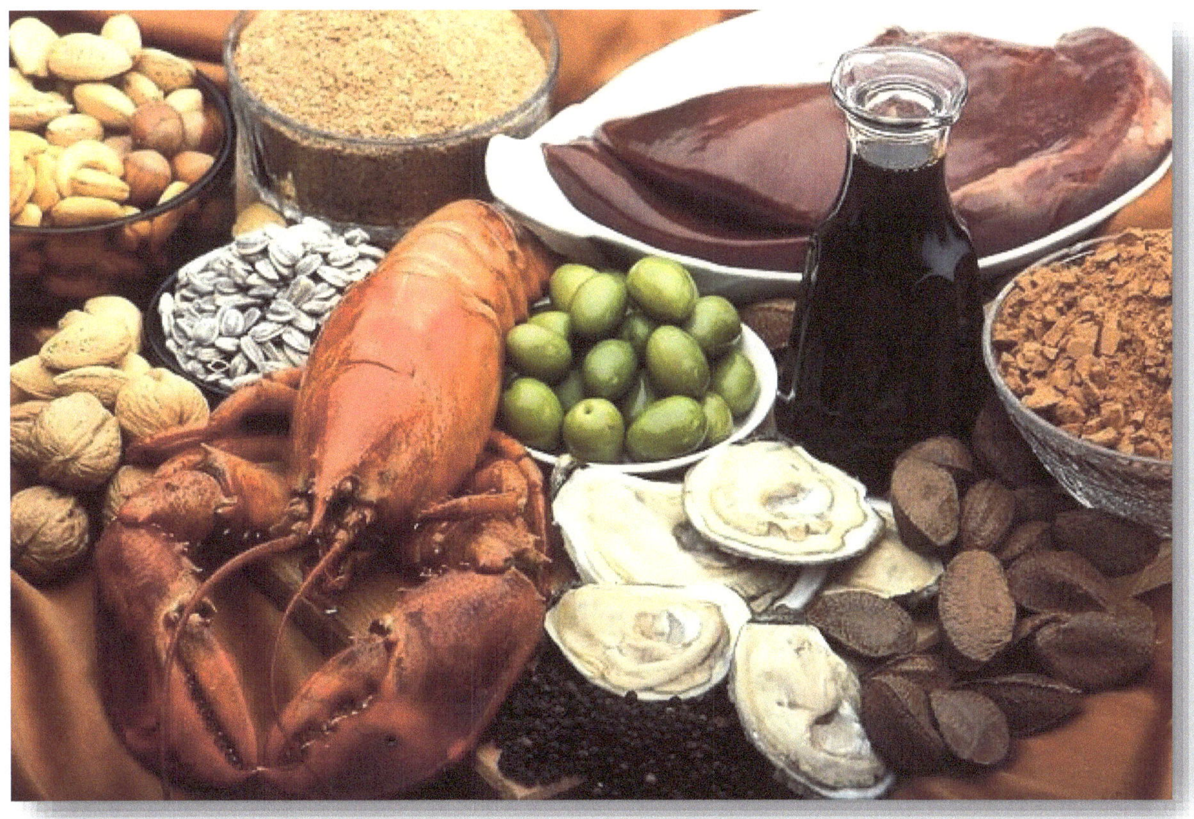

It's important, especially at first, to weigh your foods and keep track of your macronutrients (carbs, fats and proteins) so you can be sure you get into a state of ketosis. Although you can purchase test strips over the counter, they haven't proven to be very accurate, and there are other ways to reasonably determine if you are in ketosis.

Why Follow Both Diets at The Same Time?

Because intermittent fasting is more about **when** you eat and the ketogenic diet **what** you eat, both these diets go hand-in-hand and work synergistically to amplify your results when done together. First of all, it will help you avoid some of the side effects of ketosis, like the "keto flu" which can happen when your body is shifting from glucose to ketone production. (This isn't really a flu or infectious illness – just the symptoms can make it feel like it is).

It's a great way to kickstart your keto diet as a way of eating and really get into the swing of things.

When you change your way of eating to keto-approved foods, when your window to eat on intermittent fasting comes around, you have plenty of foods to eat and don't feel like you aren't going to get enough to eat. In fact, you may even have trouble getting in all your macros in the beginning.

Another huge reason people might opt for both is when you are eating keto friendly foods, you get full and stay full, thus snacking isn't a real issue. When you are fasting, it's easier to forget about eating because you aren't even hungry.

Your mental clarity is on point, your body feels sated and your energy levels are high – all while losing weight and feeling great!

It's crucial to consider your overall health and discuss your thoughts with your primary care provider before making any drastic changes to your way of eating.

The benefits of intermittent fasting and the ketogenic diet are incredible alone and magnified when combined. It takes a little discipline in the beginning, but the results far outweigh any sacrifices!

Will Ketosis Happen Faster with Intermittent Fasting?

You bet it will! Think about it. If you are restricting carbs, you are already "fasting" on a metabolic level. This forces the ketone production because you're going to need energy, and if this can be supplied from your unwanted fat stores, it is a win for you!

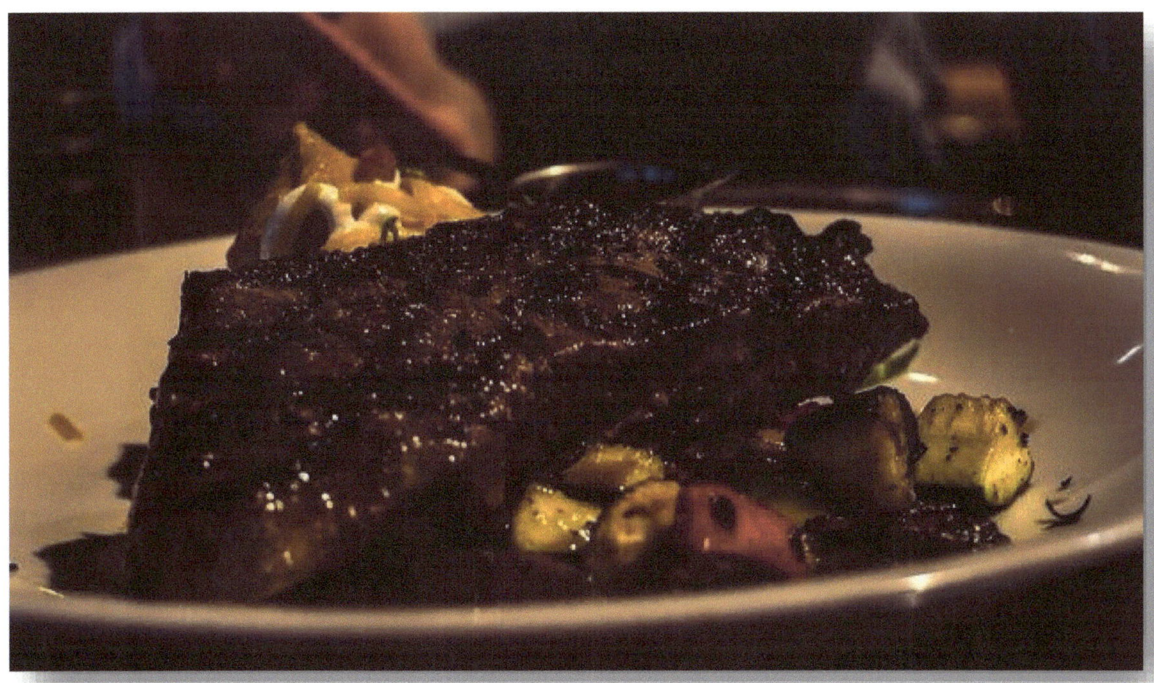

It basically mirrors an intermittent fasting routine, but on a higher level. When your body runs out of available glucose, there's no choice but to switch over to the better, more efficiently modulated fuel – stored fat.

And because it's going to be quite a few hours before you eat, your body turns into a fat-burning factory. While you are fasting, your body is busily pushing ketones so fatty acids can be broken down and used to power all of your organs, especially the super-hungry human brain.

It's an incredible cycle on a cellular level, but because this isn't an anatomy and physiology lesson, we will keep it simple. When you start an intermittent fast you are going whole-hog, all at once, and your body responds quickly.

You aren't going to feed your body every 4-6 hours like a normal diet so it has to counter your play by engaging in ketone production. Using the ketogenic diet alone, we generally reach ketosis in 48 hours, sometimes longer.

Intermittent fasting essentially jump-starts the commencement of ketosis.

Of note, glucose will forever be the preferred source of fuel for your body. If you slip up, and it happens to everyone at one time or another, and go over your carb limit for the day, you might throw your body out of ketosis.

Don't lose heart. Get back up, dust yourself off and start over.

The good news is if you're using intermittent fasting to get back into ketosis, it's not going to take long!

Other Health Benefits of Intermittent Fasting

Intermittent fasting can have many health benefits besides weight loss. Research has shown that intermittent fasting can improve your risks, and also help to prevent, against multiple diseases, including type 2 diabetes and cardiovascular issues.

Fasting has also been shown to slow down the aging process, which usually excites a lot of people. It has also been shown that fasting may help improve mental health, cognitive function and reduce oxidative stress.

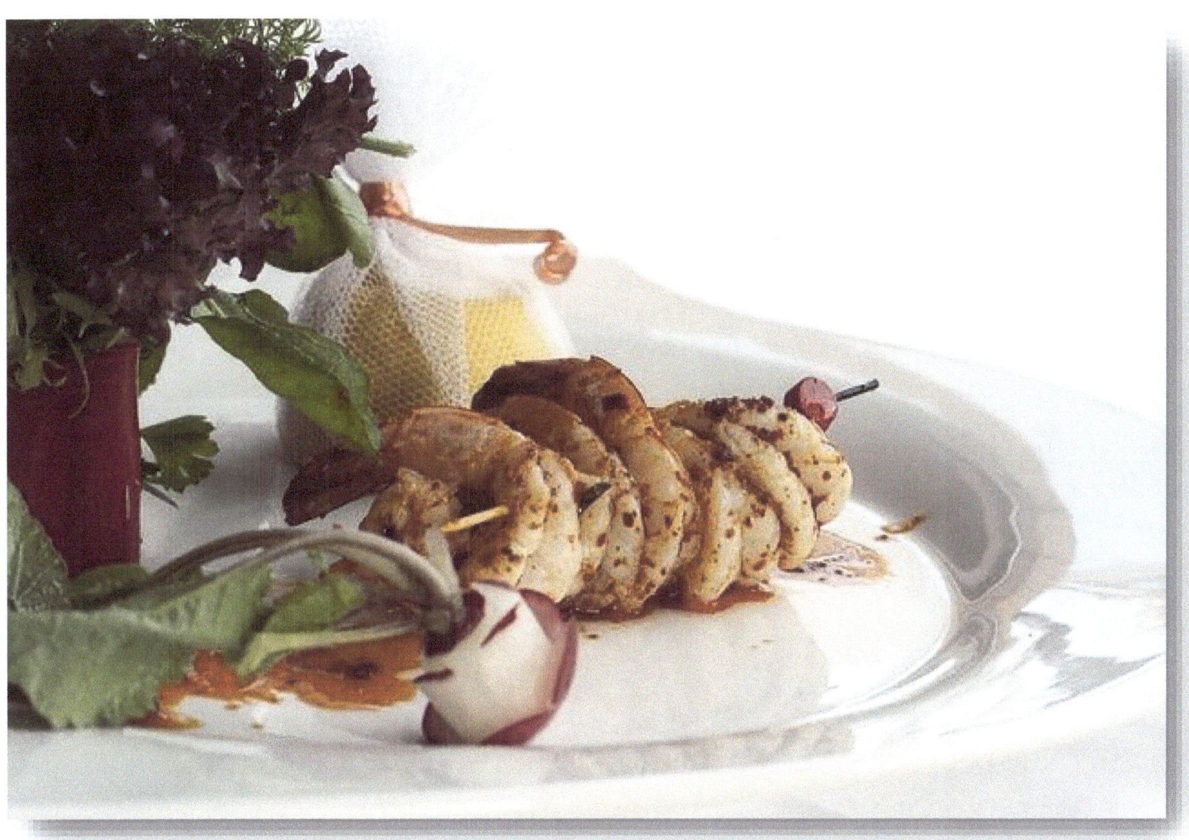

Intermittent fasting or IF has taken the health and dieting world by storm over the past few years, with more and more followers sharing their remarkable journeys to improved weight loss. While many people try intermittent fasting to help shed excess pounds, others use it because of its health benefits or because of how it helps to simplify their lifestyle.

But what is intermittent fasting, and what exactly does it do to your body and mind? Those and many more questions are answered in this beginner's guide to fast and healthy weight loss with intermittent fasting. We explore the ins and outs of this way of eating, including what science tells us about how IF can help you lose weight, live longer, and think more clearly.

Understanding Intermittent Fasting

Intermittent fasting is basically a way of eating that requires you to go for more extended periods between eating and to consume food only within a prescribed, shorter window of time. There is no specific eating plan with IF, and you can use it with any type of meal plan, including keto, whole-foods, clean eating, or whatever floats your boat. Because it is not about WHAT foods you eat, it is not a traditional diet but could be looked at to improve your eating habits, no matter what you consume.

There are many variations to intermittent fasting, which we explore more in-depth below, but the most common window is referred to as 16:8, which means 16 hours of fasting while eating all your food for one day in an eight-hour window.

Fasting has been used across cultures for various purposes for thousands of years. While some types of fasting are forced, because of a lack of food, others are performed as a part of religious or ceremonial rituals. Our ancient predecessors were often without food during the hunter-gatherer phase of our evolution, so our bodies are conditioned to go without food for extended periods. It is only within the more abundant 20th century that people in our country began to expect and assume food to be available to them several times per day.

Our bodies would argue that fasting is more natural and optimal for its function than eating three or four times per day, and those who practice IF would agree. Many who choose this way of eating report improvements in their health beyond weight loss, and they continue to adhere to a fasting schedule long after they have reached their goal weight.

Getting Started with Intermittent Fasting

There are many ways to use intermittent fasting, and you may have to try a few before you discover which works best for you and your body. The basics of IF involve splitting each day or week into periods of eating and fasting.

During fasting times, you consume only beverages that do not contain any calories or through your body out of the autophagy (cell recycling) phase. For most people, this includes water, black coffee or tea, and small amounts of bone broth. There are many arguments about how much you can eat or drink and still remain in this phase of cellular repair, but for beginners, your best bet is just not to eat anything.

Common Intermittent Fasting Methods

- **16:8 Method**- Restrict your eating to an 8-hour period each day, such as from noon- 8 pm. You can adjust your window to your lifestyle. For example, those who rise at 6 am may want to break their fast earlier in the day and quit eating before evening. You may eat two or three meals within your window as you wish. You can adjust the window slightly, with some preferring to fast for 14 hours and others for 20.
- **5/2 Method**- Restrict your eating two days a week to between 500-600 calories and eat normally the remaining five days. Some find this harder than others or experience slower weight loss.

- There are no research studies on this specific type of IF schedule, but it does fall in line with other types of fasting in terms of caloric restriction.
- **Eat-Stop-Eat Method**- This approach requires you to fast for 24 hours one to two days per week. You can choose to fast from dinner one day to dinner the next or from breakfast to breakfast; which is best for you is fine. You may drink non-caloric beverages, but you cannot consume solid food. Eat normally the other days of the week. Some people find a 24-hour fast to be difficult. You can ease into it by starting with a 14- or 16-hour fast and working your way up to a full day.
- **Alternate-Day Method**- This method has a few variations. It is basically fasting every other day, which can mean eating nothing at all to consuming 500 calories on fast days. Some even do 16:8 on fast days and normally eat the others. There are many studies on this type of alternating fast, which is quite effective.
- **The Warrior Method**- This diet is a variation on the 20:4 fast. Instead of eating nothing during the day, though, you consume small amounts of raw produce. During your eating window, you have one large meal. Food choices in this method are usually restricted to whole foods and unprocessed options.

Many people naturally like to skip meals or do not eat breakfast, which is a type of intermittent fasting, as well. Those with diminished appetites due to a low-carb diet, certain medications, or metabolic disorders may regularly practice IF without even realizing it. Most people have few issues adopting the 16:8 window because it fits nicely into the daily routine and you can still get plenty to eat during the eating window.

Weight Loss with Intermittent Fasting

Most people try intermittent fasting because they want to lose weight. Because you are eating fewer meals per day, you are almost surely eating less when you fast for longer periods. This reduction in caloric intake leads facilitates weight loss.

In 2013, researchers at Harvard Medical School showed that caloric restriction, such as with fasting, can increase the lifespan and improve metabolic functions in mammals, including people. This and other animal research provide a wealth of convincing evidence, but more research was needed to examine the effects of fasting on humans. In two separate reviews in 2015, researchers from Utah and Texas examined the effects of IF on humans and independently concluded that this way of eating has positive effects. These include reductions in LDL cholesterol, triglycerides, blood pressure, weight, fat, and glucose levels, all of which are associated with improved health.

Some would argue that intermittent fasting could lead to increased calorie consumption during the times when dieters are allowed to eat, but these same researchers did not find that to be true. In a systematic review of clinical trials using IF, researchers learned that IF resulted in a typical weight loss between seven and eleven pounds over ten weeks. This review showed that:

Dropout rates for IF were similar to those on a traditional diet of calorie restriction as was the final weight loss result. That means fasting may not be any easier than regular dieting, but it is as effective.

Those who engaged in intermittent fasting did not have any overall increase in their appetite, as some might expect with more extended periods of not eating.

When compared with other types of diets, intermittent fasting is just as effective at reducing weight and has comparable results for long-term maintenance.

Other studies have shown more dramatic results, though. For example, a 2014 study examining the effects of IF on patients with Type 2 diabetes showed that participants lost significantly more weight with intermittent fasting than with other types of dieting. They were more likely to lose belly fat, which is an indicator of improved health and lower risk for chronic disease, as well.

A 2018 study, published in *Nutrition and Healthy Aging*, found that obese people who adhered to the 16:8 protocol at about 350 fewer calories per day and lost three percent of their body weight in 12 weeks. Other researchers have examined alternative fasting schedules, as well. In a recent study in *The American Journal of Clinical Nutrition*, researchers found that obese patients who had unrestricted eating for five days followed by two days of significant caloric restriction lost more weight than those who had calorie restrictions every day. After one year, though, the results for the two groups were the same.

So, how does IF help you lose weight? And are there other health benefits or drawbacks to this way of eating? Let's take a closer look at how fasting affects the body and the mind.

Health Benefits of Intermittent Fasting

There are numerous studies indicating that fasting can improve metabolism and delay the effects of aging on the human body. Fasting does not just change how much you eat; it changes how your body processes food for energy, and it can even influence how your brain functions over time.

Effects of Fasting on Hormones and Cells

Fasting results in several effects on the body at the cellular level. For example, fasting leads to improved insulin sensitivity, which can help you keep your levels of insulin lower.

This drop can promote better burning of stored body fat, according to a 2005 study. In addition to helping your body use glucose and insulin more effectively, fasting boosts your production of human growth hormone (HGH). Higher levels of this hormone, according to The New England Journal of Medicine, is associated with an increase in lean body mass and a reduction in adipose tissue, also known as belly fat.

These two hormonal influences can help increase your ability to burn fat, which can lead to improved weight loss. But that is not where the benefits of fasting end. When you fast, your cells move into a state of repair and rejuvenation, including recycling damaged cells and forcing the death of old and dysfunctional ones. The phenomenon of cellular repair, as noted by researchers from California in 2010, results in healthier, more energetic cells being left behind, which can help you live longer.

Related to aging, fasting also can lead to changes in how specific genes related to longevity function. Researchers at the University of Chicago discovered in 2013 that fasting helps to prevent cancer as well as slow the growth of tumors. A 2006 study from Aging Research Reviews noted that fasting led to improved brain function and less neurodegeneration associated with aging.

Effects of Fasting on Heart Health

According to a 2007 study, alternate-day fasting, a form of intermittent fasting, was shown to reduce markers of inflammation in the body. Inflammation is a driving factor behind many chronic diseases, including heart disease. Researchers in Turkey noted similar effects, including a reduction in many biochemical risk factors associated with cardiovascular disease. Additional research in 2009 and 2013 further illustrated that fasting improves your heart by lowered LDL cholesterol, triglycerides, blood glucose, and inflammatory markers that are known to contribute to poor heart health.

Effects of Fasting on the Brain

Not only can fasting help your body, but it also can help improve your brain health. Intermittent fasting, for example, is associated with a reduced risk for developing neurodegenerative diseases such as dementia, according to a 2007 study. Part of these effects are due to the reduction in weight and protection against diabetes, both of which increase your chances for developing these diseases.

But intermittent fasting also helps to protect against degeneration at the neuron level. One 2003 study showed that IF helps protect brain cells from neuronal death. Researchers from The Scripps Research Institute also discovered that short-term fasting boosts autophagy in the brain, which is the process of accelerated death and recycling of damaged cells, which facilitates new cell growth.

Intermittent fasting can help boost your memory, too. A 2009 study showed that older participants were able to improve their recall of words after just three months of IF eating. And, intermittent fasting can help with mood disorders, such as depression, according to a study published in Psychiatry Research.

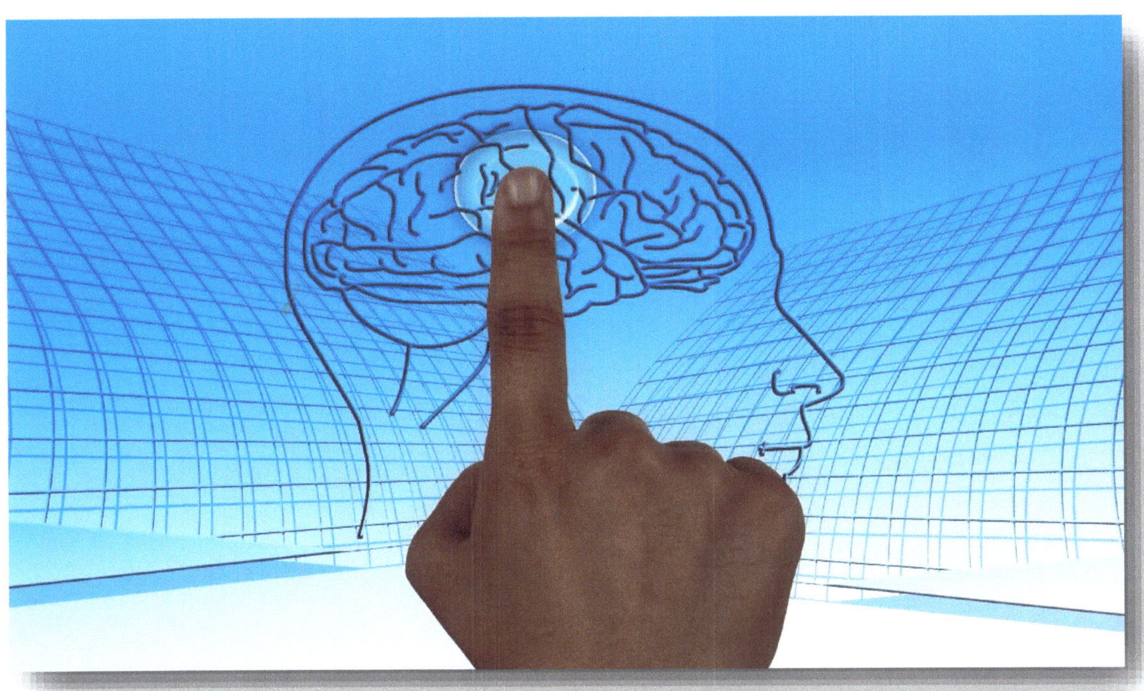

Effects of Fasting on Stress

Maintaining healthy habits can be difficult, and healthy eating takes time to plan and prepare meals. When you use intermittent fasting, it simplifies your life and allows you to focus on other aspects of your lifestyle for more significant portions of your day.

When you do not have to prepare and clean up after so many meals, you have more time to devote to other aspects of your life, which can reduce your stress level and help you enjoy life more. Many people find that fasting leads to them thinking or worrying about food less, which can help them focus on other parts of their health.

Tips for Getting the Most from Your Intermittent Fast

So, have decided to try intermittent fasting! Great!! If you want to get the most from your fasting experience, including successful weight loss, then there are a few things you can do to stay on track and make your experience more enjoyable. Here are the top tips for maximizing your benefits from intermittent fasting.

- Stay hydrated. You should still be drinking plenty of fluids, especially water. Other good options include herbal tea, sparkling water, or black coffee in moderation. Be sure you are drinking throughout the day.
- Make your calories count. Fasting is not permission to go nuts during your eating window. You should be eating healthy, nutrient-dense foods. You need plenty of fiber as well as healthy fats and protein. Since you are eating less, everything you put in your mouth should be good for you and full of nutrients.
- Eat for volume. Foods that are low in calories but high in volume will fill you up without adding to your waistline. Vegetables, fruits with lots of water, and popcorn are examples of these types of foods.
- Avoid processed foods and added sugars. When you break a fast with high-calorie foods with lots of sugar or carbs, you will immediately raise your blood sugar and probably feel bad.
- Take it slow. Start small and work your wat up to more extended periods of fasting. You may need to move your eating window in small increments until you get it where you want it. Give your body time to adjust, and you will be more likely to stick with it.
- Pay attention. Become more observant of your body, how hunger makes you feel, the effects of longer periods of fasting, and how certain foods influence you. The more you pay attention, the more informed choices you can make. Because you are eating for less of the day, you can afford to devote more time to how eating makes you feel.

It takes time. Not everyone adjusts easily to fasting. Give it time. If this is something you want to use to lose substantial amounts of weight, then it will take a while, so do not let the first few weeks of adjustment scare you off.

- Expect setbacks. We all have ups and downs. It is part of the process. What you can learn from your setbacks is more important than having them.
- Distract your mind. When you find yourself thinking about food a lot, find ways to occupy your mind until your next eating window. Engage in a hobby, go for a walk, or talk to a friend.
- Take a rest day. When you find that life is getting in the way, take a break from fasting for a day and eat as you usually would. Then, get back on track the next day.
- Find a plan that works for you. There are so many ways to fast intermittently that your experience may be completely different from someone else's. That's okay. You do not need to have the same schedule as anyone else. Figure out what is best for you. Adjust as you need. What is important is that you are comfortable, and you are getting the results you want.
- Learn the difference between boredom and hunger. Often, we eat because we have nothing else to do or because we are avoiding things we do not want to do. Learn to identify genuine hunger during your fasting periods. How does it feel in your stomach? How does it feel in your brain? Eat when you are actually hungry, and you will enjoy better health overall.
- Find support. If others in your life do not understand or agree with your decision to use intermittent fasting, just do not talk with them about it. Find support in other ways. There are many online communities devoted to this way of eating, and there are local groups in most communities that can offer you support, too.
- Try it for a month. If you are not sure if IF is right for you, try it for at least 30 days. When you are not fasting, adopt a low-carb diet, which can help reduce your cravings.

If you are not seeing the results you want or are still struggling with it after a month, decide if you are going to adjust or try something different.

- Eating windows are not for binging. Fasting works because it restricts calories. If you eat 3,000 calories during your eating window, you will not lose weight. You need to eat a healthy diet, no matter when or how often you eat.
- Focus on the quality of your experience. It is not about the destination; it is about the journey.
- Exercise in moderation. Some people, especially when they are transitioning to IF, struggle with exercise. Be sure you are eating at times that are conducive to your exercise periods, to ensure you have enough energy for your workouts.

Intermittent fasting works well when it is intermittent. You cannot fast all the time. You must be flexible with your eating and make it a part of your routine. It should not become a source of stress in your life. If it is, then it is time to move on.

Precautions and Side Effects

IF is not for everyone. Those with a history of disordered eating or who are underweight should not be using intermittent fasting. If you think this may be right for you, you should discuss it with your doctor or eating counselor first. Fasting is a form of controlled eating, which can lead to or worsen eating disorders in some people.

Women may not enjoy all the same benefits from IF as men. Some women may struggle more to lose weight or improve insulin sensitivity than men. For some, menstrual irregularity is a side effect of fasting. If you have concerns about your fasting results or side effects, you should discuss them with your doctor.

Intermittent fasting is meant to be practiced part of the time. That means you should still be eating throughout the day or week. You will not enjoy the best results if your fast is too often or too long.

If you are not getting enough sleep due to a physiological problem, you may have trouble with fasting. Those who over-exercise will also likely struggle with this way of eating.

Do not take supplements or medications that dull the appetite to sustain fasting windows. If you cannot make it through a fast without support, then the fast is too long for your body.

If you notice that you become obsessed with or consumed by eating during your eating periods, you should stop using IF. Intermittent fasting is also not a way to help compensate for making poor food choices the rest of the time.

Pay attention to how your body responds to fasting. You should stop fasting if you notice dramatic changes in your sleep quality, your energy levels, your emotional health, your hormonal levels, or your appearance. All of these are signs that IF may not be the right choice for you.

Side Effects

Most people experience hunger while fasting, which is normal. In the beginning, you may also feel weak and experience brain fog. These symptoms should lessen as you adjust to fasting.

If you have a medical condition of any kind, you should talk with your doctor before trying IF. This is especially important if you have diabetes, struggle with blood sugar regulation, or have low blood pressure. Certain medications may not respond well to fasting.

If you are trying to conceive, are pregnant, or are breastfeeding, you should avoid fasting.

Understanding the Keto Diet

You can't read a health or lifestyle blog or walk down an aisle in the grocery store these days without the words "keto diet" catching your eye. The low-carb/high-fat approach to eating has taken the country by storm and is creating quite a buzz for its ability to help you lose weight and burn fat. IF you are considering a keto diet, then it is essential you learn not only the basics but the details about this approach to eating so that you can make the best choice for you.

In this section, we explore everything you want to know about ketogenic eating, including what you can and can't eat for ketosis. We explore the health benefits as well as the precautions you should know, and we share some tips to help you make the most of your keto diet experience.

The ketogenic or keto diet is a healthy-eating plan that focuses on eating low-carb, high-fat foods. In addition to helping some people lose weight, it has other health benefits. The focus on the keto diet on low carb eating encourages your body to enter a state of ketosis, wherein it is using stored fat cells in your body for energy rather than the carbohydrates in your diet. Ketosis cannot be attained when there are already carbs for your body to use because it will use them first if available and choose to use stored bodyfat second. However, the body is more efficient when burning bodyfat than it is carbs.

Looking at the basics of the keto diet, you want to strive for limited carbohydrates and more of your calories from fat. While we each process and metabolize food differently, the most common percentages touted among the keto community today is you should keep your intake of carbs under 50 grams per day, but stricter adherents recommend eating under 30 grams per day. Most people on a keto diet strive to eat 60 to 70 percent of their calories from fat, 15 to 30 percent from protein, and just five to ten percent from carbs.

There are, however, several variations of the keto diet that you may want to consider, based on your needs. Some people do better with a cyclical keto diet, which includes five days of following a standard keto diet and two days of higher carb eating.

Other people choose to add in more carbs around workouts or physical activities. Some people believe that more protein is beneficial for them, so they choose a ratio that includes about 60 percent fat, 35 percent protein, and five percent carbs. There is little evidence to support the weight loss effects of some of these forms of ketogenic eating, as only the standard and higher protein versions have been much studied in the scientific literature.

Most of the people choosing to adopt a keto diet these days are doing so to lose weight. This type of eating plan is used under exceptional circumstances to manage specific medical conditions, such as epilepsy, but in general, it is not recommended that you follow a keto lifestyle for extended periods. Below, we explore some of the health benefits, but there is little evidence as to the long-term effects on eating for ketosis.

The ketogenic diet was initially developed to treat epilepsy and other types of seizure disorders. The ketones and decanoic acids produced by this way of eating both help to minimize seizures. Those who adhere to this eating plan, though, often experience weight loss, though. Eating carbohydrates provide your body with a ready source of energy, which means your cells never turn to your stored fat to help it perform its daily functions. Carbs also trigger cravings, which can lead to overeating, another source of weight gain.

As the buzz about the keto diet grew, more and more celebrities started following it, which caused it to catch fire among the general population. For many, eating the "keto way" is easy to follow and makes sense, which allows them to accomplish their weight loss goals.

One of the reasons that the keto diet often works, though, is that by merely focusing more intentionally on what you eat, you are more likely to eat less. People on any diet tend to reduce their caloric intake, at least for a while. Eating fats and proteins leads to feeling fuller faster, which can stop you from overeating, too. It also takes more energy for your body to process these macronutrients, versus carbs, so you are also burning more calories during digestion than you previously did.

Most people on the keto diet lose between one and two pounds per week if they follow the plan carefully. Everyone is different, though, so you should not expect your results to be the same if your metabolic rate is slower or faster.

Your caloric needs may also differ if you are an athlete, perform physical work of any kind, or spend a lot of time outdoors. Keto eating will not help you lose weight if you are still eating too many calories. Reducing your intake is still necessary for the keto diet to result in weight loss.

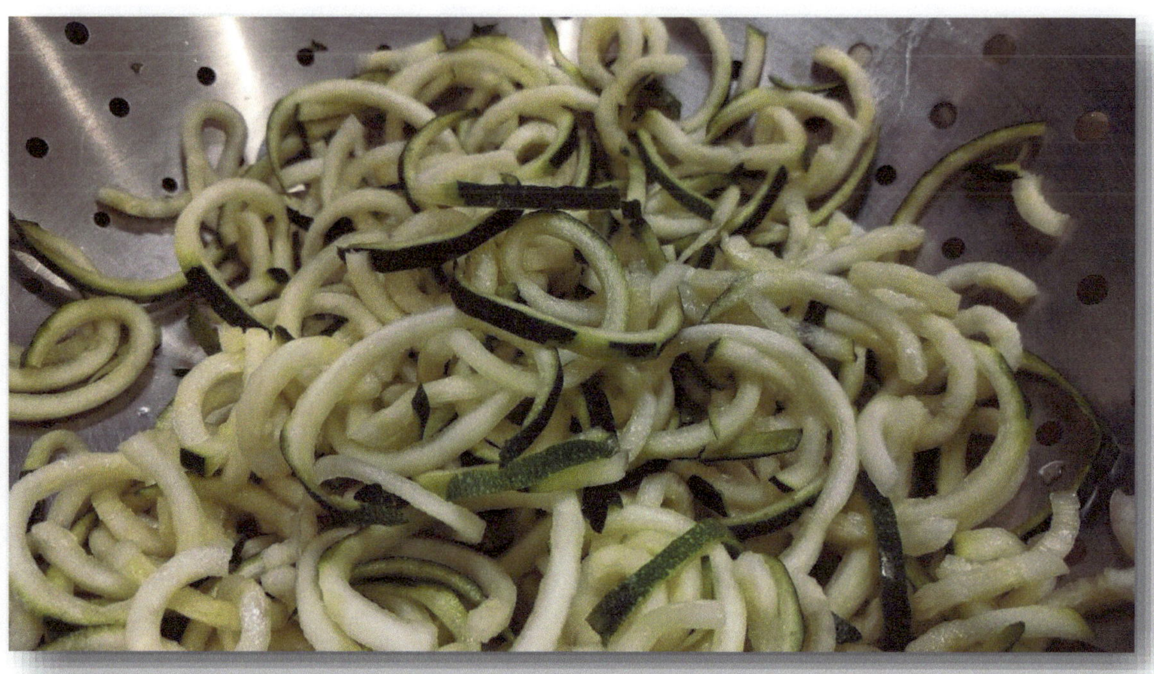

The Health Effects of the Keto Diet

In addition to helping people lose weight in the short term, ketogenic eating has been shown to help with other health problems or to improve specific conditions. For example, ketogenic eating plans help people improve their insulin sensitivity, which can help with Type 2 diabetes and prediabetes as well as metabolic syndrome.

By helping you to lose body fat, which raises insulin resistance, you can improve your glucose regulation. Those who can lose weight with ketogenic eating often experience improvements in their blood sugar and other diabetes symptoms.

The keto diet was created to help those with seizure disorders, and it is still known to be highly effective at reducing these symptoms. New evidence suggests that ketogenic eating may also help with other brain disorders and injuries, including Parkinson's disease, Alzheimer's disease, and traumatic brain injuries.

Other early research also includes some evidence that keto eating is connected to several reduced risk factors for heart disease, it is currently being tested in treating several types of cancer, and it may play a role in polycystic ovary syndrome as well as acne. These findings are all very early and require additional research to support these claims, though.

There is little research on the long-term effects of eating for ketosis. Those using this diet to lose weight should transition to a lower-fat eating plan once they have reached their weight loss goal.

The Side Effects of the Keto Diet

Many people who start a ketogenic diet experience what is known as "the keto flu," which happens when your body is transitioning into ketosis. During the first few weeks of this eating plan, you may feel as though you have the flu, including having aches and pains, a headache, brain food, and problems with your digestive tract.

As your body adjusts to using fat versus carbs for energy, you may feel like you have little energy or lack the ability to think clearly, and this time can also affect your sleep.

While these effects are temporary, they can be enough to for some people to shy away from this diet during this phase. If you want to minimize the impact of the keto flu, you can start by transitioning to fewer and fewer carbs for the weeks leading up to your transition to keto eating. It is also crucial that you drink lots of water throughout your keto experience.

Some people also experience what is known as "keto breath" when the body is transitioning into ketosis. This unpleasant odor has been compared to stale garlic and is a byproduct of your body learning to burn fat instead of carbs for energy. This, too, will pass after a time.

Many people suffer from headaches, especially at the beginning of the keto diet. You can minimize these by drinking plenty of water and getting enough electrolytes, and these headaches are mostly from dehydration.

Your body will be creating more urine on the keto diet, so you need to ensure you are replenishing your water and mineral stores regularly. In a section below, we offer more tips on how to improve your experience on the keto diet as well as maximize your chances for weight loss success.

What to Eat on a Keto Diet

So, what does one eat on a keto diet, anyway? Instead of focusing on high-carb foods, you want to center your meals on healthy fats, lean sources of protein, leafy greens, and plenty of non-sugary liquids. Unless you are also doing intermittent fasting you do not have to limit when or how often you eat on the keto diet, so snacks are allowed, too.

Healthy fats are those that are high in a variety of fats, including some saturated and some unsaturated varieties. These fats come from natural sources and are not highly processed. Examples of sources of healthy fats include avocados, whole eggs, fatty fish, nuts, chia seeds, extra virgin olive oil, coconut oil, and full-fat yogurt.

Many people think that a keto diet means avoiding vegetables, but that is false. While you want to stay away from starchy vegetables, like corn, you still need the fiber, vitamins, and minerals that are found in non-starchy vegetables. Leafy greens and cruciferous vegetables should be a part of your keto diet. These will also help to replenish your electrolytes, which can help with dehydration.

Protein sources that are rich in healthy fats and come from whole foods are also welcome in the keto diet. Grass-fed meats like beef or free-range chicken as well as oily fishes like salmon are all excellent choices.

To make things simple, we have compiled a list of keto-friendly foods below. These should comprise the vast majority of what you eat daily.

- Nuts and seeds- chia seeds, flaxseed, pumpkin seeds, walnuts, almonds, and hazelnuts
- Nut butter - made with just nuts and no other artificial ingredients or added sugars
- Eggs - pasture-fed eggs are higher in omega-3 fatty acids
- Butter and cream- grass-fed options are higher in healthy fats
- Cheese - unprocessed cheeses made with full-fat milk

- Tofu
- Meats - grass-fed red meats, poultry, sausage
- Fatty fish- tuna, trout, mackerel, and salmon
- Avocados
- Oils - avocado, coconut, and olive oils
- Non-starchy vegetables - tomatoes, onions, peppers, leafy greens, cruciferous vegetables
- Condiments - herbs, spices, pepper, small amounts of sea salt

Snacking on keto is allowed, if they fall within the nutrient guidelines of the plan. Some examples of popular keto snacks include:

- Cheese
- Nuts or seeds
- A hard-boiled egg
- A smoothie of plant-based milk, nut butter, and cocoa powder
- Yogurt mixed with nut butter
- Celery with guacamole

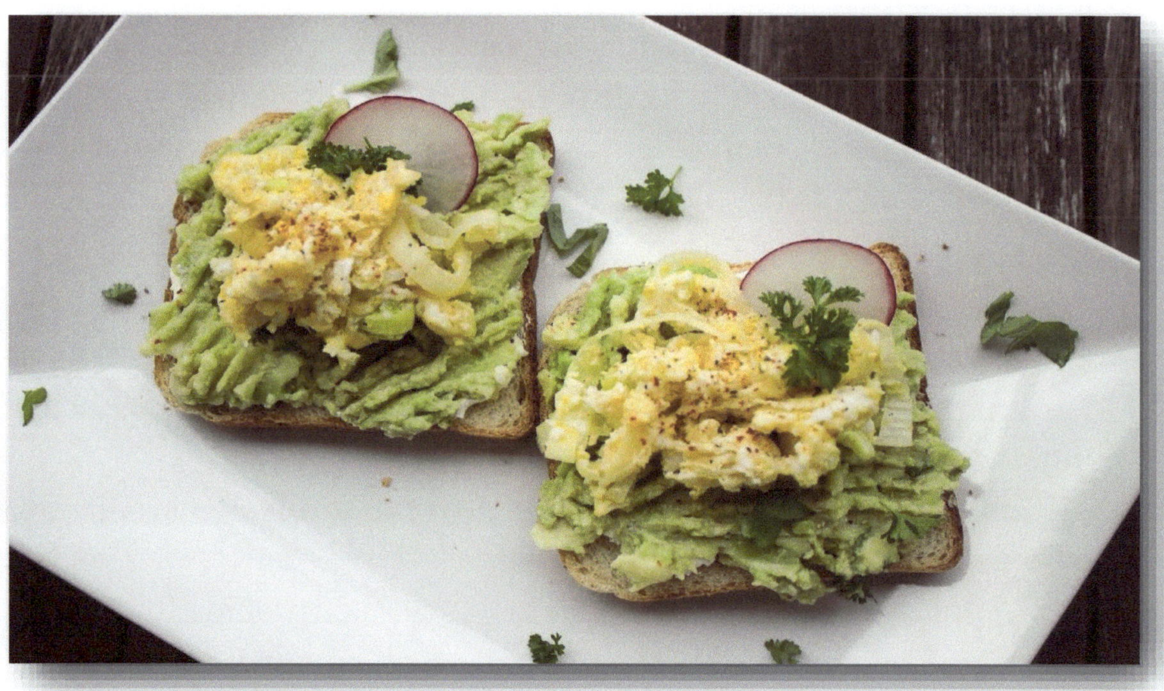

Foods to Avoid While Eating for Ketosis

While eating for ketosis, you want to avoid foods that are high in carbs. Since some people are not sure what that means or which foods are high-carb choices, the following list includes many of the foods that should be avoided on the keto diet,

- Grains of any kind, including pasta made from wheat, rice, cereal, breads, and baked goods
- Fruit should be avoided except for small portions of berries
- Beans and legumes like lentils, chickpeas, peas, and kidney beans should be highly limited in their consumption
- Root vegetables like potatoes, sweet potatoes, carrots, and turnips
- Alcohol, which is high in carbs
- Any product labeled "low fat" or "diet," as it likely contains added sugars and is highly processed
- Products marked as "sugar-free," as they often contain artificial sweeteners that can affect ketosis and are highly processed
- Foods high in sugar or with added sugars of any kind (including natural sugars)
- Most condiments and sauces contain added sugars and unhealthy fats

A Sample 7-Day Keto Meal Plan

There are literally hundreds of keto meal plans available online, and following these can help you stay on track, at least until you get the hang of what keto eating looks and feels like. Below, though, we share a typical one-week meal plan to help you envision what a low-carb, high-fat eating plan will cover.

You want to eat a wide variety of foods so that you are getting nutrients from any different sources. All foods provide specific health benefits, so eating the same thing all the time can lead to deficiencies and health problems. We have included meals only but remember that snacks are allowed as long as they fall within the nutrient guidelines of ketogenic eating.

Day 1

- Breakfast- Eggs fried with bacon, onions, and mushrooms
- Lunch- A grilled burger patty with cheese, avocado, and salsa
- Dinner- A salad of leafy greens topped with grilled steak and a hard-boiled egg

Day 2

- Breakfast- Plant-based milk with nut butter and a small handful of strawberries, blended
- Lunch- Seafood salad with avocado and olive oil
- Dinner- Parmesan-crusted chicken breast, steamed broccoli, salad of leafy greens

Day 3

- Breakfast- Omelet with ham, cheese, and spinach
- Lunch- Turkey and cheese rollups with almonds
- Dinner- Salmon and kale sautéed in coconut oil, steamed veggies

Day 4

- Breakfast- Yogurt with almond butter
- Lunch- Burger patty with cheese, side salad
- Dinner- Stir-fried pork with vegetables in coconut oil

Day 5

- Breakfast- Omelet with cheese, topped with salsa and avocado
- Lunch- Celery with guacamole, nuts, cheese
- Dinner- Pesto chicken and broccoli, side salad

Day 6

- Breakfast- Ham, eggs, and grilled tomatoes
- Lunch- Chicken salad with feta cheese and avocado oil
- Dinner- Grilled salmon and asparagus topped with butter

Day 7

- Breakfast- Omelet with cheese and vegetables
- Lunch- Leafy greens with deli ham, blue cheese, avocados, and olives
- Dinner- Baked halibut with broccolini served with butter

Supplements to Consider with the Keto Diet

On a keto diet, it is not necessary to take supplements, but many people find them to be useful for getting the nutrients they need. For example, if you are struggling with dehydration, you may want to take electrolytes or mineral supplements to ensure you are getting all that you need on this eating plan.

Many of the magnesium-rich foods that you may typically eat, such as beans and fruit, are also high in carbs, so those on the keto diet have less of an opportunity to get magnesium naturally in their diet. Taking a magnesium supplement can help avoid deficiency, which can affect your mood, energy level, and much more.

Some people on the keto diet choose to take MCT oil supplements, which stands for medium-chain triglycerides. These types of fats are metabolized differently than long-chain triglycerides, which are the type most commonly found in food. MCTs enter your bloodstream more quickly and become a source of energy much faster, which is why some people choose to take them to up their fat intake.

Adding salt, including sea salt, to your food can increase your mineral and electrolyte intake. Ketogenic eating changes your water and mineral balance, so you want to be sure you are getting enough.

Some people opt for an omega-3 supplement, especially those who do not like to eat fish, which is a significant source of these healthy fats. Those on a keto diet need to balance their omega-3 and omega-6 intake to maintain a healthy ratio, and taking a supplement can help. Most people do not get enough omega-3s in their diet.

Those who experience digestive problems on the keto diet may want to consider taking digestive enzymes. The high-fat content of this eating plan can cause nausea and diarrhea in some, but digestive enzymes can restore balance to your digestive system and help you feel better.

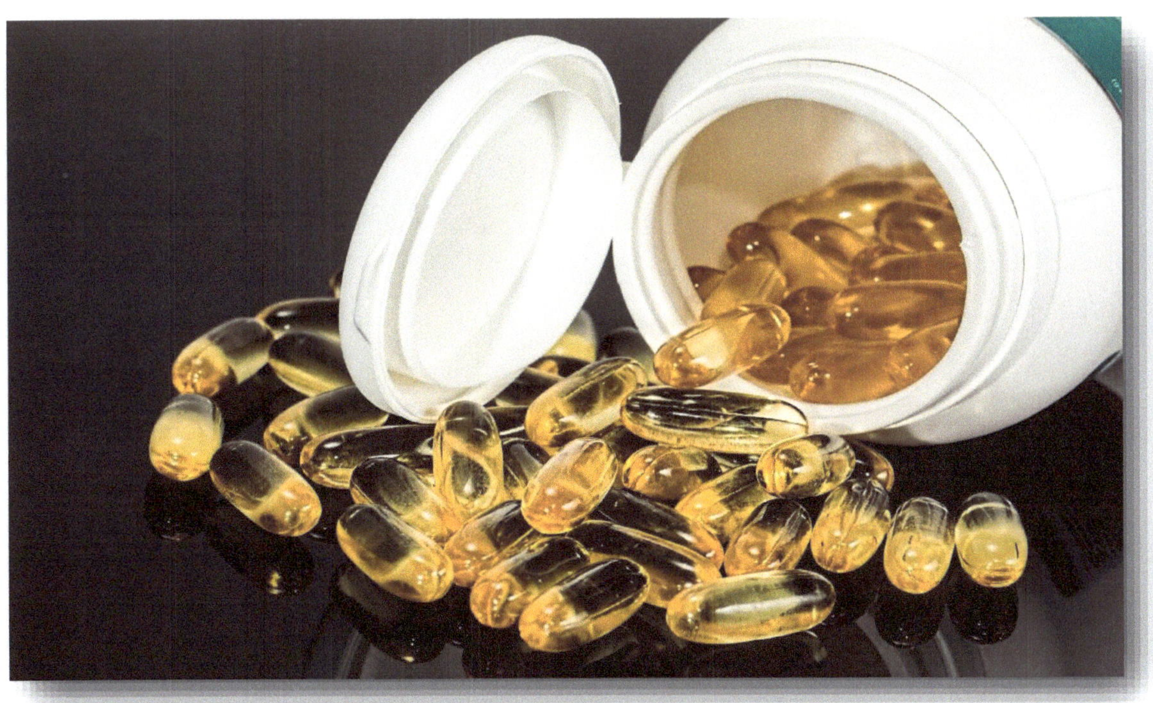

Tips for Making the Keto Diet Work for You

If you are ready to take the plunge and adopt a keto diet, there are some things you can do to improve your chances of success as well as your weight loss results. The following suggestions come from many adherents to this way of eating who have been through the process themselves. Learn from the successes and failure of others with these strategies for making keto dieting work for you.

Drink Plenty of Water

Dehydration is quite common on the keto diet, as your body is processing fluid differently now that you are no longer eating as many carbs. You will urinate more while on this way of eating, which means you are losing more electrolytes. Drink plenty of fluids, including coconut water, which is rich in electrolytes. You can also combat mineral loss with bone broth, by putting salt on your foods, and by eating water-rich plants, like celery and cucumbers.

Avoid Processed Foods

Some people look at keto as an excuse to eat whatever high-fat foods they want, but this will not help you lose weight. Adopting a cleaner, whole-foods approach is a safer, healthier, and all-around more balanced approach to eating for ketosis.

Whole, unprocessed foods like fish, avocados, and eggs will give you more of the healthy fats you need and less of the refined oils and unhealthy fats you do not. Keto is not an excuse to start eating all the fried and processed foods you can, and if you do, you will be missing out on significant nutrients your body needs.

Be Sure to Eat the Right Kinds of Fats

It is possible to eat the wrong kinds of fats on the keto diet, which can adversely affect your cholesterol levels. Unsaturated sources are best, with only small amounts of saturated fats from natural sources. Stick to the fat sources listed above for best results and avoid refined oils and trans fats at all costs.

Stock Up on Keto Staples

Any eating plan will have better results when you are prepared with the right essentials. Having a well-stocked pantry and refrigerator ensures that you are always ready to make a meal or snack that is aligned with your nutrition goals.

A keto pantry looks remarkably similar to a standard one except that that carb-rich foods have been eliminated or significantly downsized. You will not find a shelf of pasta and rice, for example, but instead will find more coconut and olive oil.

To ensure your keto success, here are some items you should always have in stock.

- Coconut oil
- Avocado oil
- Olive oil
- Ghee
- Grass-fed butter
- Eggs
- Cheeses made from whole-fat milk
- Grass-fed beef
- Cold-water fish
- Almond flour
- Herbs and spices

- Himalayan pink salt
- Coconut water
- Leafy green vegetables
- Canned tuna
- Olives
- Garlic
- Onions
- Nut and seed butters
- Balsamic vinegar
- Assorted nuts and seeds (keep in the freezer to maintain freshness)
- Various broth bases or prepared broths

Watch Your Sugars

Sugar is not a part of the keto diet in any form. This includes natural sources of sugar like maple syrup, agave or rice syrup, or honey. Many advocates of ketogenic eating also suggest avoiding other sweeteners, including stevia, monk fruit, and xylitol, at least for the first 30 days of ketosis.

When you cut all sweet things from your diet, you can better control cravings for carbohydrates. Sweeteners can often trigger binging or overeating in those with a sweet tooth. Once you have eliminated sugar for one month, you can try to introduce these healthy sweeteners in moderation to see how they affect your ability to maintain your eating habits.

One reason to avoid processed and prepared foods on the keto diet is that virtually all will have added sugars of some kind, especially those created to be "low fat" or "lite." Added sugars go by many names on a label, which is why it is important to read nutrition facts carefully to see the carbs a product contains.

Watch for Long-Term Effects

Many people feel very energized and healthy while on the keto diet, so much so that they decide to make this way of eating a long-term habit. But, keto eating for life is not recommended for everyone. If you have reached your weight loss goal, it is best to discuss your diet with your doctor to determine if staying on it longer is the right choice for you. More doctors recommend eating this way for only up to six months, perhaps longer in cases of extreme weight loss needed. Certain medical conditions may also support longer-term keto eating.

Beyond weight loss, though, staying on a keto meal plan may not be the right choice for you. Your doctor will be able to suggest if keto, a modified approach to keto eating, or some other meal plan is the best choice for you and your health.

Eat Only When Hungry

You do not need to eat frequently or at pre-determined intervals on the keto diet, unlike other eating plans. Instead of worrying about how long you should go between meals, start listening to your body. Learn to identify the signs of hunger and eat only when you feel hungry.

Eating too much or often can influence your weight loss efforts. The longer you stay on the keto diet, the more you may notice that your appetite diminishes. This is due to your decreased intake of carbs, which are natural appetite stimulants.

Pay Attention to Your Body's Signs

Some people complain of persistent fatigue while on the keto diet. This is a sign that you may not be fully in ketosis or that your body is not utilizing the fats and ketones efficiently. Try lowering your carb intake even further, and revisit everything you are eating and drinking to look for hidden sources of carbs.

You can also try adding an MCT supplement to see if that helps. If you are still experiencing this feeling after several weeks, you may want to transition to another way of eating or talk with your doctor.

Athletes May Not Benefit from Keto

Athletes, especially those who compete at an elite level, may struggle to get the appropriate nutrients with the keto diet. It can be hard to maintain or build muscle when you are not eating much protein. Those who exercise a lot or lift weights may need to increase their protein intake to achieve their athletic outcomes.

Check with Your Doctor

Before starting any new eating plan, it is always recommended that you talk to your doctor. Anyone who has liver or kidney disease should not follow a ketogenic eating plan, as it can interfere with your health. If you have gastrointestinal issues or have difficulty processing fats, keto may be hard for you to follow.

Anyone who has had their gallbladder removed should avoid this way of eating. If you are pregnant or breastfeeding, talk with your doctor before switching to a keto diet.

Those who are following the keto diet to manage a medical condition, such as epilepsy, should be working with a dietician or nutritionist, who should be monitoring their health and progress.

Tips on Eating Out with the Keto Diet

Many restaurants today cater to those who are on the keto diet, and choosing a keto-friendly option is becoming easier all the time. You can always opt for a meat or fish entrée that is not breaded or fried.

You can replace high-carb sides like pasta with vegetables. You can also opt for breakfast dishes like eggs or omelets, adding in cheese, vegetables, and meats like bacon.

To make other options keto-friendly, you can opt for burgers without the bun, add vegetables to dishes in place of potatoes, and add meats and cheeses to salads. For dessert, look for cheese options instead of sweets.

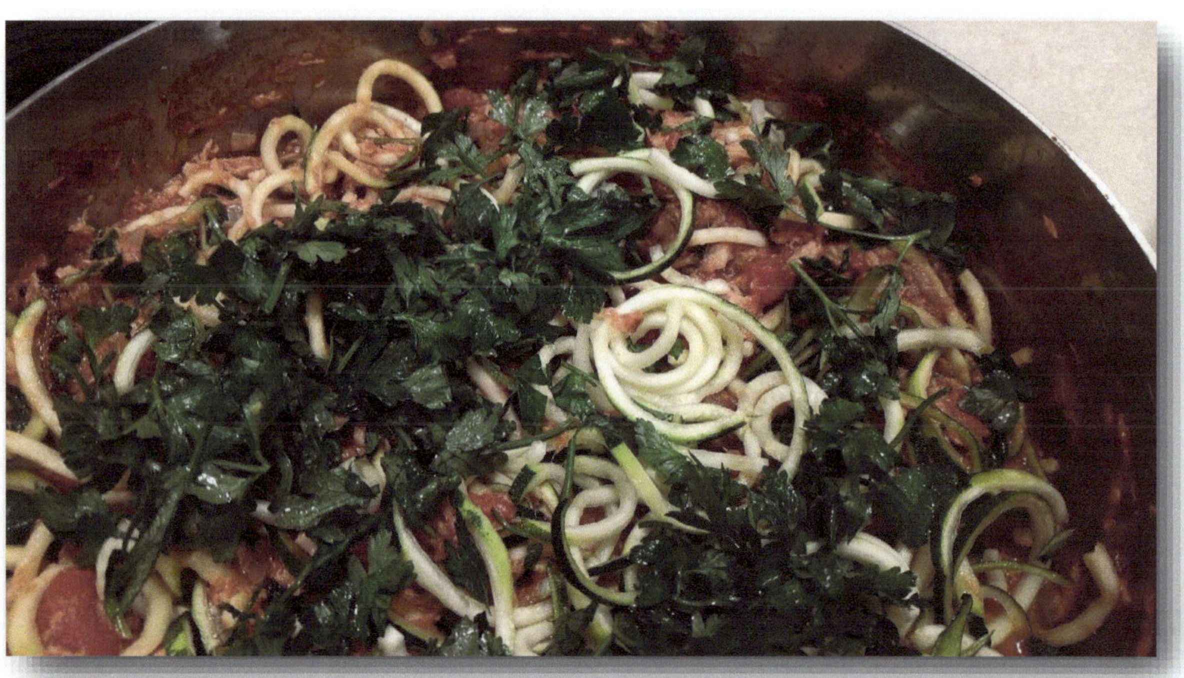

Final Thoughts

Intermittent fasting is not a diet but instead is a schedule of when to eat. The benefits of fasting have been recognized for thousands of years, as it was often practiced in conjunction with religious rites because it provides clarity to the mind.

Many people today enjoy fasting as a way to enhance weight loss. In addition to helping burn fat and decrease your weight, intermittent fasting can also provide you with other health benefits. These include better heart health, improved hormonal regulation, enhanced brain function, and less stress.

There is no one "right" way to fast. Each person must find the fasting window that works best for their needs. The most popular method is the 16:8 ratio, which allows you to eat for up to eight hours each day. Others find that a longer window of fasting works best for them, while still others choose to fast on some days but eat normally on others.

What is most important about IF is that you find a method that works for you and you pay attention to your body's needs, whether you are fasting or eating. Eating more nutrient-dense foods that are lower in calories will provide your body with the nutrition it needs while still helping you lose weight.

There are plenty of tips and tricks to use when participating in any type of fast. Staying hydrated is one of the most important factors of getting through your fast. Just because you don't eat, doesn't mean you don't drink! It is the only thing that you should and *must* consume during the fasting period.

Focusing on the quality of your food and not consuming high carb, calorie-laden foods is vital if you want to stay in ketosis and therefore lose weight, and also to help stay at your target weight when you decide to stop fasting.

Finding a ratio of fasting that works for you is the best way to achieving your weight loss goals. Learn and recognize your limits and when enough is enough, stop.

Overall, fasting can be a lot simpler and easier to stay on than your average calorie counting diet. It's still good to watch what you eat, and high calorie foods are pretty easy to spot and avoid. They're usually the processed foods or sugar-laden ones.

Simply keep clear of those types of foods and shop in the healthy aisles. Then you won't have the need to record the calories and be constantly checking the nutritional labels.

Intermittent fasting is not for everyone although it is a great diet for weight loss and highly beneficial for many people. If you want to start fasting but are not sure if it is suitable for you, first speak to your doctor or nutritionist.

When you do, they may be able to steer you to the fasting method that will most improve your chances of success.

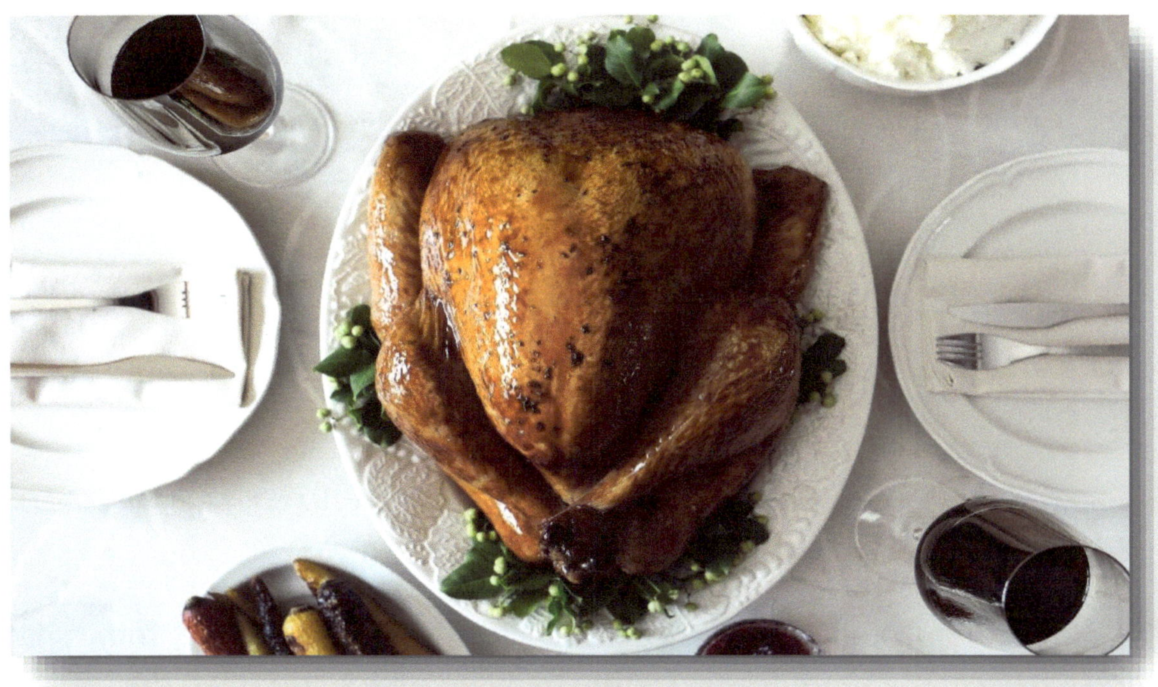

About the Author

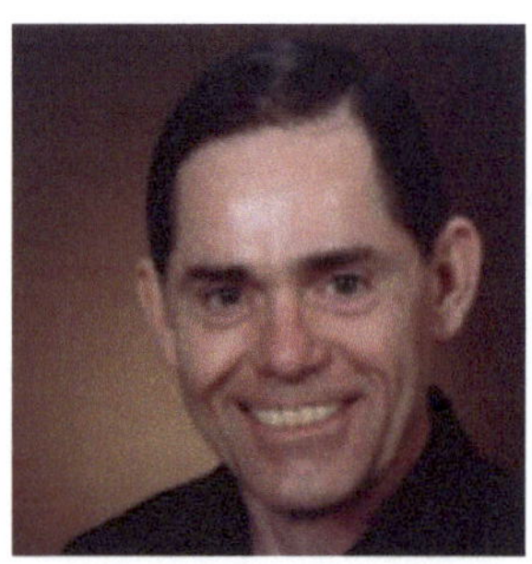

I have published numerous books on Amazon for Kindle and other publishing platforms. Both in electronic and POD formats.

While most of my books are on health and fitness in general, my topics of interest are leaning more toward aging baby boomers and the older population.

Besides my own writing, I also ghostwrite ebooks, books, reports, articles, blogs and do Kindle conversions for clients on a variety of topics. For a complete list of books, go to https://www.amazon.com/Ron-Kness/e/B0072M6PYO.

Today my wife and I are retired from our careers and live in San Tan Valley, AZ. I now write as a retirement business where you'll find me happily sitting in my office typing away on my laptop as I work on my next book or ghostwriting project . . . that is if we are not traveling on a cruise ship - our new-found mode of travel.

www.ingramcontent.com/pod-product-compliance
Lightning Source LLC
Chambersburg PA
CBHW040136240726
48664CB00002B/501